CANCER DIET COOKBOOK FOR NEWLY DIAGNOSED

Delicious Recipes and Guidance for Your Cancer Journey

Dr. Rachel Ferguson

TABLE OF CONTENTS

Contact Us:

You can also contact us in our 24hrs email address for guidance or advice.
mailto:drrachelferguson@gmail.com

Reach out below to see more of our health books and lots more in our store!

Drrachelferguson

Appreciation

We would be forever grateful if you could take a few moments after you've finished reading, to leave us a positive review on Amazon. Your review will not only help us to reach a wider audience, but it will also help other readers to discover the value of our book. We know that your time is valuable, so we truly appreciate your willingness to share your thoughts with us. Thank you in advance for your kind review.

Dear cancer patients,

In the face of this challenging journey, I want to offer you words of encouragement and support. You are not alone in this fight, and your strength and resilience are truly remarkable. Here are some words to uplift and inspire you:

Stay Strong: You are stronger than you realize. Every day that you face this battle with courage and determination, you demonstrate incredible strength. Keep pushing forward, even on the toughest days, because you have the power to overcome.

Embrace Hope: Hold onto hope tightly, for it is a guiding light in the darkest of times. Believe in the possibilities that lie ahead, in the potential for healing, and in the advancements of medical science. Let hope be your fuel for resilience and perseverance.

Celebrate Small Victories: Remember to celebrate every milestone, no matter how small. Each step forward, each moment of relief or progress, deserves recognition. Find joy in the little triumphs and let them motivate you to keep fighting.

Lean on Your Support System: Reach out to your loved ones, friends, and healthcare team. They are here to support you emotionally, physically, and mentally. Allow them to be a source of comfort, encouragement, and strength throughout your journey.

Practice Self-Care: Take care of yourself holistically. Listen to your body and rest when needed. Engage in activities that bring you joy, whether it's spending time in nature, practicing mindfulness, or pursuing hobbies that uplift your spirit.

Seek Moments of Joy: Amidst the challenges, look for moments of joy and happiness. Surround yourself with things that bring you laughter, beauty, and peace. These moments can provide respite and remind you of the beauty that life still holds.

Express Your Feelings: It's okay to feel a range of emotions during this time. Allow yourself to express your fears, frustrations, and concerns. Seek support from therapists, support groups, or online communities where you can connect with others who understand your journey.

Find Inspiration: Seek out stories of survivors and individuals who have triumphed over cancer. Their journeys can inspire and uplift you. Draw strength from their experiences and use their stories as a reminder that you too can overcome this obstacle.

Take it One Day at a Time: Remember that healing is a gradual process. Take each day as it comes, focusing on the present moment rather than overwhelming yourself with the future. Celebrate the progress you make, no matter how small.

You Are Resilient: Cancer may test your resilience, but it cannot break your spirit. You have the power to rise above this challenge and come out stronger on the other side. Believe in your ability to overcome and never lose sight of the fighter within you.

You are not defined by cancer; you are defined by your incredible strength, courage, and resilience. Keep fighting, stay hopeful, and know that there is an entire community of individuals supporting and cheering you on. You are not alone in this journey, and together we stand with you, united in hope and solidarity.

INTRODUCTION

Mary's life changed when the doctor told her she had cancer. Her life was abruptly flipped upside down as she fought to accept her diagnosis and the upcoming course of therapy. She couldn't help but feel anxious about what was ahead as she waited in the waiting room for her first chemotherapy visit.

Mary was confident she would do all she could to combat the illness. A nutritious diet would be essential to her rehabilitation since she had always believed in the power of food. But when she dug more into her investigation, she discovered that the data was confusing and overwhelming. What food is best for her? What is to be avoided?

That's when she saw a need for a cookbook created especially for those who had just received a cancer diagnosis—a cookbook highlighting the science behind how food may treat sickness and offering delicious and healthy recipes. As a result, Mary set out to write the "Cancer Diet Cookbook for Newly Diagnosed," a comprehensive manual for consuming healthfully while receiving cancer treatment.

Mary discovered from her studies and experience that a balanced diet might be pretty effective in the battle against cancer. She wrote this book intending to empower people to take control of their diet and maximize their chances of healing.

It is impossible to exaggerate the value of food for cancer patients. Chemotherapy and radiation therapy are two cancer therapies that may be hard on the body, making it harder to fight the illness and raising the risk of consequences. A nutritious diet may give the body the energy and nutrition needed to heal and recover while supporting the immune system.

A nutritious diet may aid in managing the adverse effects of cancer therapies and bolster the body's immune system. For instance, certain meals might assist with nausea relief, while others can aid in preventing constipation.

A nutritious diet may also aid in preventing the emergence of other medical issues that can make treating cancer more difficult.

For instance, it has been shown that eating a diet rich in fruits and vegetables lowers the risk of heart disease and diabetes, two conditions often co-occurring with cancer.

Noting that there is no one-size-fits-all diet for cancer patients is crucial. Each patient will have different nutritional demands depending on the kind of cancer, the stage of the illness, and the type of therapy being taken. However, the nutrition and energy required to support the body's battle against cancer may be found in a diet high in whole foods, including fruits, vegetables, whole grains, and lean meats.

The Science of Diet and Cancer

Cancer and nutrition have a nuanced connection, according to research. While food cannot treat cancer, it may be vital in halting its progression and assisting the body's battle against it.

First, certain nutrients are necessary for cancer cells to develop and multiply. These nutrients may be obtained via a sugar- and processed diet, aiding cancer formation. On the other hand, a diet high in plant-based whole foods, such as fruits, vegetables, whole grains, and legumes, may provide the body with the nutrients it needs to combat cancer and maintain general health.

Second, a nutritious diet may aid in lowering bodily inflammation, which has been connected to the onset and spread of cancer. Berry, leafy greens, and fatty salmon are foods strong in antioxidants and anti-inflammatory substances that may aid in decreasing inflammation and guard against cancer.

Thirdly, a robust immune system may help fight cancer. This is made possible by a good diet. Vitamin C, zinc, and other immune-supporting elements are found in foods that may assist in bolstering the immune system and the body's capacity to combat cancer cells.

While nutrition may be a crucial ally in the body's battle against cancer, it should not be used as a replacement for medical care; it is vital to remember. A thorough treatment plan for cancer patients should be created in collaboration with their medical team and include dietary and medicinal therapies.

Nutritional needs for cancer patients

Focusing on a patient's dietary requirements is critical since cancer and its therapies may influence their nutritional state. Here are some essential vitamins and minerals that people living with cancer may want to pay attention to:

Protein: Since muscle mass might be impaired after cancer therapy, protein is crucial for preserving it. Lean meats, fish, poultry, eggs, dairy products, and legumes are all excellent protein sources.

Calories: Cancer therapies may raise a patient's energy requirements, and malnutrition might result from not getting enough calories. To maintain or increase their weight if they are losing it, patients should try to eat adequate calories.

Vitamins and minerals: Taking meals high in these nutrients is essential since specific vitamins and minerals may be more difficult to absorb during cancer therapy.

For instance, patients may need to concentrate on eating foods high in vitamin D, calcium, iron, and B vitamins.

For cancer patients, staying hydrated is crucial since several medications might make you dehydrated. Water, herbal tea, and low-sugar electrolyte drinks are among the fluids that patients should try to consume in large quantities.

Fiber: Since constipation is a frequent side effect of cancer therapy, it's essential to have adequate fiber in your diet.

Foods to Stay Away From When Treating Cancer

Even while cancer patients must concentrate on eating a balanced, nutrient-rich diet, there are certain items they may need to restrict or stay away from while undergoing treatment. Here are a few instances:

Raw or undercooked foods might raise the chance of contracting a foodborne infection, which is risky for cancer patients with compromised immune systems.

Dairy products that have not been pasteurized: Dairy products that have not been pasteurized might also increase the risk of contracting a foodborne disease. They may be especially risky for individuals receiving chemotherapy or radiation treatment.

Meat that has been processed or cured, such as bacon, sausage, and deli meats, may contain a lot of salt, nitrates, and other potentially dangerous ingredients.

Foods heavy in sugar and fat may be inflammatory and encourage cancer formation.

Alcohol: Alcohol may weaken the immune system and raise the chance of developing several malignancies, including breast and liver cancer.

How to Create a Healthy Plate

For cancer patients, creating a healthy plate is crucial because it may assist in ensuring that they are receiving the nutrients they need to support their health and recovery. The following advice will help you create a nutritious plate:

Vegetables and fruits should comprise half of your plate since they are rich in vitamins, minerals, and antioxidants that may help prevent cancer and promote general health. Try to fill your container with various fruits and vegetables, both in color and kind.

Pick lean proteins: Lean proteins, including those found in fish, chicken, and lentils, may aid in recovery and the maintenance of muscle mass. Thin meat slices are preferred over processed meats.

Include entire grains: entire grains may provide fiber and other crucial nutrients. These grains include whole wheat bread, quinoa, and brown rice, as examples. Instead of choosing refined grains with fiber and minerals removed, try to pick whole grains.

Limit your intake of saturated and trans fats since they may cause inflammation and accelerate cancer development. Select wholesome fats like those in nuts, seeds, and fatty fish.

Watch your portion sizes: gaining weight might harm cancer patients if you overeat. Consider using smaller dishes and plates, and watch your portion amounts.

Keep yourself hydrated: Cancer patients should be hydrated since specific therapies might dehydrate them. Throughout the day, try to consume a lot of fluids, such as water, herbal tea, and electrolyte drinks, with little to no added sugar.

Tips for meal planning and grocery shopping

For cancer patients, meal preparation and grocery shopping may be difficult, particularly if they suffer side effects from their therapy. Here are some suggestions to make grocery shopping and meal preparation easier:

Spend some time preparing your meals and snacks for the next week. This helps you avoid hasty judgments that might not be the best.

Please list the items you need to purchase for the next week and stick to them when you go grocery shopping. By doing this, you can make sure you have everything you need to prepare nutritious meals and snacks and prevent making impulsive purchases.

Shop the perimeter: You can often locate fresh vegetables, lean meats, and whole grains outside the supermarket.

Limit your processed and packaged goods purchases and concentrate your shopping in these store sections.

Stock up on nutritious staples: Make sure your cupboard contains healthy foods like whole grains, canned or frozen fruits and vegetables, lean meats, veggies, and whole grains. When you are short on time or energy, this might help you quickly assemble a nutritious supper.

Cook in bulk: If you prefer to avoid cooking one day, cooking in bulk may save you time. A large quantity of soup, stew, or chili might be a good idea to prepare in advance and freeze for later use.

Convenience meals, such as pre-cut fruits and veggies, may be helpful when you have limited energy. However, use convenience foods cautiously. Just read labels carefully and choose products low in added sugars and salt.

Feel free to ask relatives or friends for assistance with food shopping or meal preparation. They could be delighted to help you, which might relieve some of your burden.

Recipes for breakfast

For cancer patients, the following breakfast dishes may help them get their day off to a good start:

Yogurt parfait with berries:

Ingredients:

- 1 cup of Greek yogurt, plain
- Strawberry, blueberry, and raspberry-filled 1 cup of mixed berries
- 14 cups of granola
- 1 teaspoon of honey

Instructions:

- Yogurt and honey should be blended in a small dish.
- The berries should be combined in a separate dish.
- In a glass or dish, layer the yogurt, berries, and granola.

Enjoy!

Egg and avocado toast:

Ingredients:

- 1 whole grain bread piece
- Mashed avocado, half
- 1 egg
- Pepper and salt as desired

Instructions:

- The bread is toasted.
- Toast is covered with mashed avocado.
- In a nonstick pan over medium heat, fry the egg until done to your taste.
- On top of the avocado toast, place the egg.
- Add salt and pepper to taste.

Dispense and savor!

Nuts and Berries in Oatmeal:

Ingredients:

- Oats rolled in a cup
- 1 cup of the milk or water of your choice
- Strawberries, blueberries, and raspberries totaling 1/2 cup
- 1 tablespoon of chopped nuts (walnuts, pecans, or almonds)

Instructions:

- In a small saucepan, heat the milk or water to a rolling boil.
- Turn the heat to low and stir in the oats.
- Stirring regularly, boil the oats for 5-7 minutes or until they are tender and the mixture has thickened.
- Add the chopped nuts and mixed berries on top.
- Dispense and savor!

These breakfast dishes are easy to prepare and provide a well-balanced mix of protein, fiber, and healthy fats to help cancer patients power the day ahead.

Smoothie, oatmeal, and egg dish recipes

Here are some recipes for smoothies, oatmeal, and egg dishes that might provide people living with cancer with a filling and delicious breakfast:

Smoothie

Banana-Oat Smoothie

Ingredients:

- 1ripe banana
- Oats rolled in a cup
- 50 ml of almond milk
- Greek yogurt, plain, in 1/2 cup
- 1 teaspoon of honey
- One-half teaspoon of vanilla extract
- 1/8 teaspoon cinnamon powder

Instructions:

- In a blender, combine all ingredients and process until completely smooth.
- Pour into a glass, and then sip.

The green smoothie

Ingredients:

- 1 serving of baby spinach
- 1/2 cup of pieces of frozen mango
- 12 cups pieces of frozen pineapple
- 50 ml of coconut water
- Chia seeds, one tablespoon
- 1/2 lime juice

Instructions:

- In a blender, combine all ingredients and process until completely smooth.
- Pour into a glass, and then sip.

Oatmeal:

Cinnamon Apple Oatmeal:

Ingredients:

- Oats rolled in a cup
- 1 cup of the milk or water of your choice
- a single, diced tiny apple
- 1/8 teaspoon cinnamon powder
- 1 tablespoon of chopped nuts (walnuts, pecans, or almonds)
- 1 tsp. of honey

Instructions:

- In a small saucepan, heat the milk or water to a rolling boil.
- Add the cinnamon, apple slices, and oats.
- Once the oats are cooked and the mixture has thickened, reduce the heat to low and simmer for 5-7 minutes, stirring regularly.
- Add some chopped nuts and honey on top.
- Dispense and savor!

Almond-blueberry oatmeal:

Ingredients:

- Oats rolled in a cup
- 1 cup of the milk or water of your choice
- 12 cups fresh or frozen blueberries
- 1/4 cup almond butter
- 1 tablespoon of almonds, chopped
- 1 tsp. of honey

Instructions:

- In a small saucepan, heat the milk or water to a rolling boil.
- Include the blueberries and oats.
- Once the oats are cooked, and the mixture has thickened, reduce heat to low and simmer for 5-7 minutes, stirring regularly.
- Add the almond butter and stir.
- Add some honey and sliced almonds on top.
- Dispense and savor!

Omelet dishes:

Scrambled Spinach with Mushrooms:

Ingredients:

- 2 eggs
- A half-cup of baby spinach
- Sliced mushrooms in a cup
- Pepper and salt as desired
- 1/9 cup olive oil

Instructions:

- Warm the olive oil in a nonstick skillet over medium heat.
- When the mushrooms have softened, add them.
- Baby spinach should be added and cooked until wilted.
- Add salt and pepper to the beaten eggs before beating them in a small bowl.
- The eggs should be poured into the pan and scrambled until done.

Vegetable omelet

Ingredients:

- 2 eggs
- Chopped bell pepper, 1/4 cup
- 14 cups finely minced onion
- 14 cups of tomato, chopped
- Pepper and salt as desired
- 1/9 cup olive oil

Instructions:

- Warm the olive oil in a nonstick skillet over medium heat.
- Cook the tomato, bell pepper, and onion until tender after adding them.
- Add salt and pepper to the beaten eggs before beating them in a small bowl.
- Cook the eggs in the skillet until they are set.
- Serve the omelet folded in half.

Appetizers and snacks

Here are some recipes for healthful and nourishing cancer patients' snacks and appetizers:

Vegetables and hummus:

Ingredients:

- 50 ml of hummus
- Baby carrots, 1/2 cup
- Sliced bell peppers in a cup
- Cut cucumbers in a cup

Instructions:

- The hummus should be put in a small bowl.
- Around the hummus, arrange the small carrots, bell peppers, and cucumbers.
- Dispense and savor!

Whole Grain Crackers with Greek Yogurt Dip:

Ingredients:

- Greek yogurt, plain, in 1/2 cup
- 1 teaspoon of lemon juice
- 1/4 tsp. dried dill
- Pepper and salt as desired
- Dipping crackers made with whole grains

Instructions:

- Combine the Greek yogurt, lemon juice, dill, salt, and pepper in a small bowl.
- With whole-grain crackers on the side for dipping.

Sweet Potato Fries Baked:

Ingredients:

- Fries made from one big sweet potato
- Olive oil, 1 tbsp
- Pepper and salt as desired

Instructions:

Set the oven to 425 °F.

Add salt, pepper, and olive oil to the fries made from sweet potatoes.

On a baking sheet, arrange the fries in a single layer.

Bake the fries until they are crispy and golden brown for 20 to 25 minutes, turning halfway through.

Dispense and savor!

Produce Salad

Ingredients:

- 1 cup of diced mixed fruit, including mango, kiwi, strawberries, blueberries, etc.
- 1 teaspoon of honey
- 1/2 lime juice
- Mint leaves for garnish, fresh

Instructions:

- In a small dish, mix the lime juice and honey.
- The mixed fruit should be combined in a giant dish.
- Over the fruit, drizzle the honey-lime dressing and toss to coat.
- Fruit salad should be served in bowls or cups and topped with mint leaves.

Almonds & Berries with Cottage Cheese:

Ingredients:

- Low-fat cottage cheese, half a cup
- Strawberries, blueberries, and raspberries totaling 1/4 cup
- 1 tablespoon of almonds, chopped

Instructions:

- Mix the cottage cheese and mixed berries in a small bowl.
- Add some chopped almonds on top.

Main Dishes

Here are some healthful and nourishing main dish recipes for cancer patients:

Salmon on the grill with asparagus:

Ingredients:

- 4 fillets of salmon
- 1 pound of trimmed asparagus
- Olive oil, 1 tbsp
- Pepper and salt as desired
- Serving slices of lemon

Instructions:

- Set the grill's temperature to medium-high.
- Olive oil, salt, and pepper are drizzled over the salmon fillets and asparagus.
- The salmon fillets should be cooked through after grilling for 4–5 minutes on each side.

The asparagus should be cooked with a little char, about 2 to 3 minutes each side.

Lemon wedges should be served with the salmon fillets and asparagus.

Stir-fry with quinoa and vegetables:

Ingredients:

- Quinoa, one cup
- 2-cups of water
- Olive oil, 1 tbsp
- 1 sliced onion
- 2 minced garlic cloves
- 2 cups chopped mixed veggies, such as carrots, bell peppers, and broccoli
- Low-sodium soy sauce, two teaspoons
- 1 teaspoon of sesame oil
- Pepper and salt as desired

Instructions:

Bring the quinoa and water to a boil in a medium saucepan. Once the quinoa is soft and the water has been absorbed, reduce the heat, cover the pan, and simmer it for 15 to 20 minutes.

Olive oil should be heated in a large pan over medium heat. Sauté the onion and garlic for two to three minutes or until tender.

The mixed veggies should be added to the pan and stir-fried for 5-7 minutes or until crisp-tender.

Add the cooked quinoa along with the sesame oil and soy sauce. To taste, add salt and pepper to the food.

Kabobs with chicken and vegetables:

Ingredients:

- 4 cubed, skinless, boneless chicken breasts
- 1 red bell pepper, chopped
- 1 yellow bell pepper, chopped

- Sliced zucchini from 1
- 1 red onion, chopped
- Olive oil, 1/4 cup
- Balsamic vinegar, two teaspoons
- 1/9 cup Dijon mustard
- Oregano, dry, 1 teaspoon
- Pepper and salt as desired

Instructions:

Set the grill's temperature to medium-high.

Chicken, bell peppers, zucchini, and red onions are all skewered together.

Mix the olive oil, balsamic vinegar, Dijon mustard, and dried oregano in a small basin.

After brushing the skewers with the olive oil mixture, salt and pepper should be added.

Once the chicken is cooked and the veggies are soft, grill the skewers for 10 to 12 minutes, turning once.

Desserts and Sweet Treats

Here are some recipes for healthy and nourishing desserts and sweet treats for cancer patients:

Yogurt parfait with mixed berries:

Ingredients:

- 1 cup of blueberries, strawberries, and raspberries mixed
- Greek yogurt, one cup
- 14 cups of granola
- 1 teaspoon of honey

Instructions:

- Combine the berries and honey in a small dish.
- Layer the Greek yogurt, granola, and berry combination in a parfait glass or Mason jar.
- Layers are added again till the top.

Dispense and savor!

Apples Baked:

Ingredients:

- 2 cored and cut-in-half apples
- Brown sugar, 2 tablespoons
- a teaspoon of cinnamon
- 1 teaspoon melted butter
- Chopped walnuts, 1/4 cup

Instructions:

- Turn the oven on to 375°F.
- In a separate dish, mix the brown sugar and cinnamon.
- The apple halves should be covered in melted butter before adding the brown sugar mixture.
- Bake the apple halves for 20 to 25 minutes or until soft.
- Serve the apples with the chopped walnuts on top.

Avocado Chocolate Pudding:

Ingredients:

- Pitted and peeled two ripe avocados
- Unsweetened cocoa powder in a half-cup
- 50 ml of honey
- 1/fourth cup almond milk
- Vanilla extract, 1 teaspoon
- A dash of salt

Instructions:

- Blend or process the avocado, cocoa powder, honey, almond milk, vanilla essence, and salt until smooth.
- Put the pudding in a bowl and refrigerate for at least one hour.
- Dispense and savor!

Oat-and-banana cookies:

Ingredients:

- 2 mashed ripe bananas
- Rolled oats, 1 cup
- (Walnuts, pecans, and almonds) 1/4 cup chopped nuts
- Chocolate chips, 1/4 cup
- Vanilla extract, 1 teaspoon

Instructions:

- The oven to 350 degrees Fahrenheit.
- Mix the mashed bananas, rolled oats, finely chopped almonds, chocolate chips, and vanilla essence in a medium bowl.
- Spoonful of the mixture should be dropped onto a parchment paper-lined baking sheet.
- The cookies should be baked for 15 to 20 minutes or until golden brown.

Dispense and savor!

Meal Planning and Preparation

Maintaining a balanced diet while receiving cancer treatment may require careful meal planning and preparation. Here are some hints for organizing and preparing meals:

Pre-plan your meals: Set aside some time each week to review the meals you'll eat that week. You can keep organized and make sure you have all the materials on hand by doing this.

Make a shopping list of all the items you need once you plan your meals. This may assist you in maintaining concentration and preventing grocery store impulsive buys.

Once a week, grocery shopping is recommended to save time and guarantee that you always have fresh items on hand.

Ingredient preparation in advance: You may prepare some elements to save time throughout the week.

For instance, you may schedule a batch of grains like quinoa or brown rice or cut up some veggies.

Cook in bulk: Consider making meals in advance and freezing them for later in the week. This may save you time and guarantee that you always have wholesome meals available.

Use simple recipes: Look for dishes that can be prepared quickly and easily. Many tasty and healthful foods may be prepared in 30 minutes or less.

Feel free to seek family and friend assistance if you are feeling overburdened by the planning and preparation of meals. They could be eager to pitch in with dinner preparation, grocery shopping, or cooking.

Conclusion

Maintaining energy, strength, and general well-being after cancer treatment depends on eating a nutritious diet. Additionally, a healthy diet helps lessen adverse effects and increase the efficacy of therapy. Various delicious and wholesome recipes are included in The Cancer Diet Cookbook for Newly Diagnosed, along with advice on planning and preparing meals. Cancer patients may design a diet that suits their unique requirements, interests, and preferences according to the advice in this book. Remember that a healthy diet is just one component of cancer therapy; for the most outstanding results, it's crucial to collaborate closely with your medical team.